GROWING UP WITH ANXIETY DISORDER

By

Mark Arthur Pagel

ISBN: 1-4033-8442-8 (e-book)
ISBN: 1-4033-8443-6 (Paperback)

This book is printed on acid free paper.

1stBooks – rev. 12/10/02

This book is dedicated with love to my Mom

and Dad

TABLE OF CONTENTS

INTRODUCTION

When I was about three years old, my parents were divorced. I live with my mom and I am always able to see my dad whenever I want. I am lucky to have two good parents, even though they are divorced. Families can include an aunt or uncle, or grandparents, or even a family friend. There are many foster families as well.

Although some people may point to my parents being divorced as a reason for my anxiety disorder, I do not believe that it is. Anxiety disorder is caused by a chemical imbalance in the brain. Nerve impulses are transmitted from one neuron to another in the brain, and anxiety disorder occurs when certain neurons in the brain get too much of a certain chemical. In other words, the nerve impulses are not transmitted equally in the brain.

It is easier to understand problems when they are VISIBLE, such as when someone has a broken arm or a broken leg. People can relate to these problems because a broken arm or leg is something that people can see and identify with easily. However, it isn't this way with a disorder in the brain because a disorder in the brain cannot be seen physically.

My mom and I moved into an apartment after my mom and dad were divorced. The neighbors seemed to come and go so quickly in this neighborhood, and that was a source of stress.

One of my earliest recollections is when I was in nursery school, which I attended only once or twice a week. My mom thought that it was a good idea to have other children to associate with because I was an only child. Sometimes I wonder what it would have been like growing up with a brother or sister, but I did enjoy the time I spent with my cousins, who were close to my age. I remember that my nursery school teacher was a caring, elderly lady. I don't recall much of my days in nursery school since this was such a long time ago. I do remember looking forward to my mom picking me up, after a few hours. I'm quite certain that many children would feel some anxiety attending nursery school, but for me it was harder because of the social anxiety disorder, which at that time it was not determined that I had. I felt more at ease at home with a babysitter than I did at school where there were more people. I felt somewhat nervous starting kindergarten in the fall of 1978.

CHAPTER ONE: THE GRADE SCHOOL YEARS

Back when I was a boy, some twenty years ago, anxiety disorder and panic attacks were not well known. Children and adults alike had them, but nobody knew what they were. Very little was known about social anxiety disorder, and it certainly was not known that a chemical imbalance in the brain was the cause of this almost debilitating mystery. Little has been written from a child's point of view on this subject; this is what I hope to accomplish with this book.

A lot of people experience anxiety. It keeps people on their toes. However, with some people, as with me, it can be overwhelming. This is what the anxiety disorder is. There are many symptoms of social anxiety disorder, now also called generalized anxiety disorder. Symptoms can include being sick to your stomach, being short of breath, being nervous when there is no need to be nervous, dryness in your mouth, sweating, and shaking. These symptoms can improve with medicine and also with deep breathing exercises. The purpose of this book is to show others that there is hope.

One of the advantages of having anxiety disorder today is that it is accepted. People are starting to understand what it is. There are even commercials for anxiety and depression today. I did not have these advantages growing up, and I would never have thought that there would be commercials for anxiety and depression. I am glad to see this progress has been made.

One of the very first incidents of anxiety at school that I can remember was when I was in kindergarten. There was a magician performing one day. The magician showed us a coin and then it vanished. She said that we should help her look for it. The class sat on small chairs and we were looking under the chairs for the coin. Finally everyone stopped looking and we sat back down. Then the magician lady said that it was right behind my ear and showed the class the coin. Now, of course, I can rationally say that it was an amateur magic trick. FROM A CHILD'S PERSPECTIVE, HOWEVER, I didn't understand what was going on. I remember thinking that I should have known where the coin was, and I also remember feeling a lot of anxiety. At the same time I wondered, "How could it be behind my ear the whole time?" After all, I didn't even feel it behind my ear. This is merely one example of the stress that I had to cope with for my entire grade school years.

I remember when I was very young my mom and I would go over to my grandma and grandpa's house and grandpa would make some good meals on the red brick grill which he had built himself. The trees and flowers in grandma and grandpa's backyard were beautiful; grandma always had a gorgeous flowerbed. I also remember having fun swinging on the swing in their spacious yard. Later, a patio would be added onto this area, but at this time there was only a picnic table by the grill. I remember grandma and grandpa had a dog, Spotty, who was a lot of fun.

I remember walking with grandpa near grandma and grandpa's property. At the end of their property there were railroad tracks for a freight train. Grandpa would always pick me up and he would run down to the end of the yard, and we would watch the train go by. I still remember the delicious meals that grandpa made on the grill: chicken, pork chops, or hamburgers. Near the picnic table was a hammock which all family members took turns enjoying. My uncle and his family would also visit on Sundays. I had a lot of good times at grandma and grandpa's house, and I had fun with my cousins who were close to my age. I enjoyed these times and I wished that I didn't have to return to school where there was so much stress.

My grade school teachers had no empathy whatsoever. They couldn't put themselves in the other person's place. When I started the first grade in the fall of 1979, I was away from home more than I had ever been, and with the anxiety this made it almost unbearable. I remember one day going up to the school and coming into the classroom and then darting right back out to the car, and coming to my mom. The teacher came outside and just stood there as if to say, "Why are you causing such trouble?"

It was extremely hard to get to school but I was able to get there, at least for a while. To make it easier to be in school, my mom put some photos in my lunchbox of the family. This did help somewhat. I would come home and watch Mr. Roger's Neighborhood, and that would cheer me up somewhat. You see, there was no medicine that I could take; the anxiety disorder was not well known. At least I could talk to my mom and dad. However, when I myself couldn't understand or define the problem, it made it that much more difficult to convey my feelings to anyone else.

Looking back now, I wish that I had told my mom and dad more of the details of how miserable I was in school. I told my mom and dad some of the incidents, but I really hadn't gone into much of the detail of the things that were happening. I would now advise children to tell specific things to their parent or guardian when it comes to school abuse or anything else out of the ordinary.

I liked talking with my grandma and I also liked talking with my grandma's neighbors. Grandma had neighbors within walking distance and I would often set out to visit them. My grandma was able to see that I was safe from her window. Grandma and I always had a good time at her house. It was at grandma's house that I first learned how to play "Scrabble" which is still one of my favorite of all board games. I think that playing "Scrabble" helped enhance my interest in writing. My grandmother would also help me with my homework.

Mom, dad, and I went to talk to a social worker but that really didn't help much. Nobody could understand why I didn't want to go to school. The fact was that I wanted an education, I just didn't want to be made fun of by my classmates. It wasn't that I didn't want to be there; I was too NERVOUS to be there. I just did not fit in at school. None of the teachers could seem to understand that. They were there for their paycheck and that was it. They did as little as they possibly could to help the students. They were so intimidating that I never spoke about these incidents, even to my mom and dad. I guess that I just wanted them to go away.

It would be nice if I could say that my classmates helped ease my anxiety, but I can't because they didn't. In fact, they made my anxiety worse. All through grade school I was picked on and made fun of.

I remember during the first grade the class would point forks at me, as if they were going to hurt me with the forks. This made me very nervous. I asked them not to do that, but once they found out that it bothered me, some of them did it even more. One time I asked my first grade teacher if I could be moved and she said angrily, "Just sit down." So I had to endure this for months.

On a brighter note, one summer my mom, dad, and I went down to Florida. Back then, only the Magic Kingdom was in Orlando. Epcot, MGM Studios, and the Animal Kingdom had not even been built yet. They were working on the tram to Epcot. I can vaguely remember one of the drivers saying, "That will take people to the new theme park." I had fun at the Magic Kingdom. I was a little nervous taking my first flight though, but I got through it and I even enjoyed it. In Florida we went to Sea World and saw the seals. This was a fun summer. I remember sitting in the "Splash Area" hoping to get splashed by one of the dolphins. I didn't get splashed but I did get sunburned! Everything turned out good though.

I didn't feel much anxiety during this vacation. My "first flight certificate" came in the mail a few days after I returned home. I still have this certificate in with my important papers.

After summer vacation, I always had to return to school, and it was always difficult. During gym class in grade school, I always wished that I would be picked first or even in the middle. Instead I was always the very last person picked. This added to my anxiety. It made me feel that I wasn't a good player even though I knew that I was pretty good. I remember feeling embarrassed, high strung, and tense. I was never in any after school activities because the anxiety prevented me from participating. Sometimes I would dream of scoring the winning basket for my team, but I was never on a team all through grade school and my classmates sure didn't let me forget it.

My classmates made a big deal about the kind of shoes I wore. I didn't wear the "In Brand" and this and that.

There was one time in the third or fourth grade that my teacher asked who did a certain thing, I said, "that wasn't me." Then the teacher said, "I didn't ask who it WASN'T, I asked who it WAS." This man was very high strung and should not have been teaching. He would speak very quietly and sometimes I wouldn't hear him. He would mumble. He had no business being in the teaching profession. He was really bad. One time he spoke so soft that I didn't hear that there was a quiz. I was drawing while others were taking the quiz. I was an attentive student and I was sitting towards the front of the class, but I still couldn't hear him. When he collected all the quizzes, he noticed that I didn't have a quiz, and he demanded to know why I didn't take the quiz. Before I could explain he yelled, "You young man are going to get a zero!" I remember that I was very very nervous. I was out of breath and I was starting to get dizzy. My throat went dry and I got very sweaty. I remember that I wanted to get up and go over to his desk and tell him that I couldn't hear him, but my anxiety held me back, and I was unable to convey my words to him. A lot of times I would come home from school and I would throw my books down and I would be almost in tears. This incident, among many others, contributed to a great deal of anxiety at school.

There was another time when this same man made another snide comment to me. I asked to go to the bathroom, saying, "Can I go to the bathroom?" He replied, "I don't know, can you?" Then I said, "May I go to the bathroom?" and he said yes, looking very annoyed. Here again I remember thinking about how nervous I was, and I was sweating. A lot of times I could hardly eat my lunch, and the kids gave me a hard time about that. One time I drew a picture of this teacher, looking angry. Another one of my classmates showed this picture to the teacher. The teacher said, "Well, what makes me angry?" I don't remember what was said after that, but the point is that I must have thought of him as a basically angry person to have drawn a picture like that. The teachers at this school had no patience at all and had no idea about how to deal with children.

Another time I remember that the second grade teacher came into the classroom and said that I wouldn't be going outside to recess because I had to practice my handwriting. I can still remember her exact words, "Prepare to do some neat penmanship." They would use big words that many of the kids didn't understand. After studying psychology for a while in my college years, I can now say that the reason they did this was to try to make the kids feel inferior because they were so insecure about themselves.

Although the anxiety was a detriment, I did have fun at times during my grade school years. One summer I went up to the Wisconsin Dells with my mom, grandma, uncle, aunt, and my cousins. We had fun up there. I also enjoyed the times we would have family baseball games in my grandma's backyard. Sometimes we would watch movies on the big screen T.V. in my grandma's basement and we would order out for pizza. These were good times. I don't want to give the impression that my childhood was complete misery. Only when I was at school did I feel that the anxiety was unbearable. When I was out in public, ESPECIALLY in the classroom, I felt the anxiety disorder get worse. For example, one summer I went to a creative writing class. Before I went in the building I stopped. After the class when I came back out to the car, my mom asked me if I thought I had forgotten something, and I said that I was just saying a prayer that I would make it through the class. I remember feeling tense in this class. There was this one girl who made fun of me, she made fun of my name. So my mom and I came up with a poem, "Showing Respect for your fellow Classmate's Name." Here It is:

"I'm very proud of my own name, and everyone else should feel the same. Making fun of someone's name is not my idea of a game. You should show respect for your fellow man, and laughing at his name should be banned. A joke is good, a joke is grand, as long as it doesn't get out of hand. Because laughing at one's name is bad, it makes the person feel very sad. We need a lesson to be taught, and everyone should give that some thought. I will feel tall as a giant about my name, and everyone else should feel the same. Don't be rude, don't you see, we can make this world a better place to be. I'd like to shout my name aloud, and that's what this poem is all about. I'm very proud of my own name!"

After I read this poem the teacher in the creative writing class said that it was good and she said, "You guys were really giving Mark a hard time yesterday." This teacher cared for her students, unlike the teachers at my grade school.

During one of my summer vacations, my mom and I went out to California to visit my mother's aunt, who is my great aunt. This helped to relieve my anxiety, but my anxiety was still there. We went to the beach with Aunt Dorothy and I saw the Pacific Ocean for the first time. I enjoyed the airplane ride. I did not have a lot of anxiety when I visited my great aunt. Even back then I enjoyed writing. I carried a notebook with me during most of my vacations, writing down the experiences, one of which was going to Disneyland. Aunt Dorothy said that she was afraid to do or say anything because it would get in my book. I laughed and, of course, I wrote that down in my notebook. We had a good time and I saw Los Angeles. Overall, this was a positive experience for me. Shortly, summer came to a close and school would be starting again.

I had a teacher at the grade school that I referred to earlier that assigned way too much homework. A lot of the kids complained but it didn't do any good. There were nights when I would stay overnight at my grandma's house. She helped me with my homework. Sometimes we were doing homework right up to my bedtime. Sometimes my grandma would watch me when my mom had to work. One night my grandma and I worked on a math assignment so long that it almost made the two of us sick. My grandma had a lot of patience and we did the best we could with the assignment. The next day I turned in the assignment and it was graded in class. The teacher said to me in front of everyone else, "Boy, when you flub it up you really flub it up." Here again, I felt nervous and self conscious. I did the best I could, and it was new material that I had never studied before. This was in the fifth grade.

There was another incident, away from school, that caused me a great deal of anxiety. I was taking the garbage out one day and the neighbors had a visitor that had a dog that was tied up to a tree in the backyard. This dog was a large German Sheppard. Since my grandma and grandpa's dog Spotty was so friendly and I had always liked dogs, I didn't think that there was any reason to be afraid of the dog.

When I went out to the backyard, the dog started to run toward me. This leash was much too long for a dog like this. I ended up dropping the garbage bag and running. The dog ran after me and bit me as I ran away. I remember being frightened by this, and once again the anxiety disorder compounded my tense feelings. For years after that I avoided dogs and after many years I finally conquered this fear.

In the fall of 1984 things really started to fall apart. A new, arrogant teacher took over the fifth and sixth grade classes. He never had control of the classroom and the kids did not respect him.

One of my classmates came home crying, her mother said. Still nothing was done by the principal. Once again I had a teacher that didn't care and still my peers were making fun of me. I let them so they knew that they could get away with it. The anxiety prevented me from standing up to them.

One time during gym class I was supposed to tumble on a mat. The teacher was getting impatient and told me to hurry up. I was a little afraid of doing the tumbling but it was part of the class that day. Finally the teacher himself pushed me on the mat. He had no business whatsoever doing that. I started coughing because I landed wrong. He took me out to the drinking fountain to get a drink of water. He said that I didn't have to do any more tumbling that day. The other kids were laughing at me in the background and calling me names. I remember thinking that it was a serious matter and that they shouldn't be laughing. How would they like it if they were in my place?

One day that same school year during lunchtime the teacher left the room. One person started making fun of me and then several others joined in. One person grabbed my popcorn and poured it over my head. That did it. I left the room to find the teacher. I told him that the kids were making fun of me and that this had been going on for many years. Then I asked him if he could talk to them. He gave me some reply like, "When you grow up are you going to go call the teacher and ask him to fight for you?" It was clear that he didn't want any responsibility. He did not care about his students at all. I believe that a grade school teacher should care about his or her students. After this incident I did not want to stay at this school. I came home and I knocked everything off of a shelf in the kitchen. I was very angry and upset. I was very nervous and the bottled up stress of this school finally came out. I transferred in the middle of the 1984-85 school year. I was twelve years old at the time.

In 1984 I took some guitar lessons. I wish that I had followed through on them. With school and the anxiety I didn't want to continue. Now, I wish that I had, but it's too late to go over that now, and if I would ever want to play the guitar I know that I could still take lessons. I still have the guitar that my mom bought me.

In my spare time I would watch television programs. Also, during my grade school years I would collect action figures. I collected Star Wars, Super Powers, and He-Man action figures. I had fun making up different storylines with my action figures. I watched the television show, "He-Man and the Masters of the Universe" after a stressful day at school. This helped my anxiety a little bit.

There were some action figures that I really had a hard time finding. I composed a letter to the company that made the toy line and I asked them if these action figures were still in production. The company wrote back and sent me seven of the ten action figures that I inquired about, free of charge! I was ecstatic and I couldn't believe it. I still have the action figures on my dresser in my room. This was something very positive during a very stressful time in my life, having just changed schools.

Another thing that I would like to add about school is that the popular kids in school such as the football players and cheerleaders should try to help kids that are not as outgoing or popular as they are, rather than try to make fun of them. I think that tension would decrease for all the kids if everyone would try to be friends and not give other kids a hard time.

Undoubtedly, everyone has their best friends, but that doesn't give anyone the right to intentionally exclude certain kids from games at recess. It also doesn't give anyone the right to treat certain classmates with cruelty.

It was January of 1985 and it was a very tumultuous time. I was glad to be rid of my old school, but now I had the anxiety about the new school. What would it be like? Would I finally have friends? I was now in a new school and I didn't know anybody. I felt very self-conscious, especially on the first day.

It was in very late February of 1985 that I saw a psychologist and a psychiatrist. They were very nice and they did help me somewhat. However, they thought that I just did not want to go to school. I really wanted to but I just couldn't. I missed a lot of days. Also, it was about this same time that I had to get glasses and that change made me even more self-conscious than I already was. So, once again, I wasn't into sports or activities and I wasn't popular.

One day my sixth grade teacher came over to our house and tried to get me to school. We talked for a while but I told him that I just couldn't go. Later I overheard him tell my mom that he wouldn't call the truant officer yet. I knew that it would come to that soon, however. I was afraid of what was coming.

Toward the end of March 1985, things were looking very bad. I was distraught. My mom was really feeling down. This whole thing was very hard on the both of us. It was really an ordeal for the both of us. Even though my psychologist and psychiatrist listened, it was not a well known fact that the problem was a social anxiety disorder, which is caused by a chemical imbalance in the brain. My mom had no other choice but to call the hospital and have me hospitalized because I had to be in school and I wasn't. I met a variety of people there. At least people weren't making fun of me. A lot of the kids were on drugs, though. They were going through rehabilitation. One girl was raped. These kids really needed help. It made me appreciate that I wasn't in their shoes. These kids were really from troubled homes and I felt sorry for them. At first, I could not leave the floor at this hospital. After a few days, however, I was able to get a pass and leave for a few hours. One day the entire floor went to a movie, under supervision. I was released in three weeks. Mom and dad visited me, as well as my grandmother. My psychologist and psychiatrist also came, and after I got out of the hospital they continued to help me.

It was June of 1985 and I needed help to finish the sixth grade. My mom found a public school teacher to tutor me, and I successfully finished that grade. It was an uphill battle with the anxiety, but I was able to finish the sixth grade. However, I had to think about getting back to school in the fall.

In the fall of 1985, even though I had an incredible amount of anxiety, I was able to get back to school. I didn't want to have happen what happened the previous spring. It was incredibly difficult. I still didn't know that I had an anxiety disorder. Changing schools changed nothing. Again, I wasn't popular with my fellow peers and I wasn't accepted at all. I wasn't on the basketball team or in any other sports. The students had someone to pick on.

During recess I would play basketball, shooting hoops by myself. I really dreaded the school day. It seemed like the time would really crawl by. I stopped and took a deep breath and said to myself it's not worth getting upset over.

My seventh grade teacher, who was also my eighth grade teacher, was a wise-cracking, know it all, arrogant man.

During the eight grade I enlisted in a forensics competition. I read a poem. I had to read it three different times to three different judges. I received a first place red ribbon for this forensics competition. I was very nervous during this competition, but with deep breathing exercises I was able to get through it and get a first place ribbon. The deep breathing does help and it can be done anywhere.

Despite all of the anxiety, I got through the eight grade.

On June 3, 1987, I finally graduated from grade school. I was so happy to finish! It seemed to have lasted forever. Now I was preparing for high school. Would it be any different? I wondered.

CHAPTER TWO: THE HIGH

SCHOOL YEARS

I didn't want wearing glasses to compound my anxiety of starting high school, I thought that finally activities and sports wouldn't matter and that I would fit in. It didn't take long for my bubble to burst and for me to realize that I wouldn't fit in no matter how hard I tried. In the fall of 1987 I started high school with a lot of anxiety. I was really on edge and tense. There was this obnoxious jerk who thought he was God's gift to the girls. All of the guys were pretty much jerks. These guys were very, very immature. The only ones who were more clueless were the girls who dated them. The 1987-88 school year was one of the worst I ever had. I felt a lot of anxiety at school. In Spanish class I remember looking at the snow falling outside and feeling sad. There was a girl I liked but I didn't have the courage to ask her out. You see, I wasn't with the "in crowd."

I tried to socialize, to no avail. Very few people seemed to want to talk to me or associate with me. This was supposed to be a well respected school. I came to realize that in this school, if you're a guy and you're not playing sports, you're nothing. That's not the way it should be. The high school years are supposed to be fun.

In February of 1988, my Mom and I went to Orlando, Florida, and we had a good time. This was a nice change. We saw all the different tourist attractions and this helped relieve my anxiety somewhat. Even on this great vacation, however, when we would go to a restaurant or one of the theme parks, I would get a little tense. This is proof that the anxiety disorder never goes away. I was even wondering to myself why I would be so nervous. After all, I was on vacation, I was away from the classroom and all the students. Why would I be nervous?

I was able to return to school after our trip to Florida and I finished my freshman year. However, I was unable to finish my sophomore year.

In my sophomore English class there were times when I felt sick to my stomach. This was a symptom of the anxiety once again. I started missing class again I was so nervous. I remember looking at the clock and thinking, "If I can just get through this class there's only one more." There was a guy in this class that made me very nervous. He must have been on drugs because he acted so crazy. He made me feel very tense because he was a very intimidating person. He was a punk. He was the worst of all the students when it came to bothering me. He would call me names, knock books out of my hands, and do anything to try to humiliate me. He never hit me though. Sometimes I wish that he had because then I would have had something concrete to report to a teacher and maybe he would have been disciplined. I tried to sit as far away from him as I possibly could during English class, and I remember wishing that the class was over. My eyes lifted to the clock again in hopes that the class was almost over. It was just too much stress for one person to handle. The fifty minute class seemed like an eternity and I could feel his presence in the room, like a ghost that you want to wish away but you can't. Looking at the clock only made the time go slower. If I could, I would erase this part of my life. It was bad.

In the fall of 1988 the stress and mental anguish was starting to wear on my physical health, and I got mononucleosis. Everything was becoming too much: the mental cruelty, nobody at school talking to me, the anxiety and tension, the name calling, the humiliation; I

47

was sick of it. I was ready to scream. I didn't think it would be like that. I thought that I'd get a break, especially after all of those bad years in grade school. The illusion of fun during my high school years remained just that, an illusion. I felt desperate. I felt sick. Sometimes I wanted to cry like I had never cried before. This was worse than grade school and there was no way out.

Because of my anxiety I never attended any high school dances, homecoming, prom, or any other activities, even though I really wanted to. I was the outcast. No matter how cool I acted I was viewed as a freak or an outsider. I was the kid who would always study, dress normal, and avoid after school activities. The more I was viewed this way, the more I withdrew. All I wanted was to fit in, but it couldn't be done at this school.

I just couldn't take all the pressure anymore. It was really getting me down, and it was wearing on my mom too. Once again I want to emphasize that children should talk to someone in their home such as a parent or guardian. I talked a little to my mom and dad, but it wasn't enough. I never went into any details. I think that I didn't want to upset them with all that was going on.

Looking back, I seemed like a different person in that school.

Whenever I left it, I was myself: friendly, relaxed, and talkative. However, when I was there, I was shy, quiet, withdrawn, and very tense and nervous. One time when I asked my biology teacher about an assignment date he replied, "You worry too much." That was really absurd.

1989 was a horrible year. My mom went on the night shift in January of that year because she wanted to be at our apartment in the morning to help me get to school.

I had a hard time just walking into the school. I remember that I stayed in the car as long as I possibly could, even when I would get there very early and it meant a long wait in the car. My Dad would drop me off in the morning and pick me up in the afternoon. I always felt a chill when I entered that school. I felt cold, very cold.

One time two guys threw my shoes around the gym when we were changing into gym clothes. I told them that I would get the teacher and then they stopped. I was wondering to myself, "What's with these guys? I'm here for an education."

Finally it got to be too much in February of 1989. I missed a lot of school due to mononucleosis. Plus I just couldn't go to school because of the anxiety. Once again, I had to get help for this problem, and still very little was known about the anxiety disorder. Our insurance was different and I spoke with the two most incompetent therapists that I ever met. One of the therapists said that I was just lazy and he told my high school that there was no reason that I should not be attending high school. He made matters worse. I tried to tell him my plight but he was just not smart enough to help. Then after a while, I spoke to the psychologist who was just as ineffective. I spoke with him and he did not help me at all.

Then my mom and I got a very threatening letter from the high school principal. In the letter he said, "Mark has CHOSEN not to attend school and with this choice comes consequences." My mom and I were so disgusted because we knew that it was NOT a choice.

I pulled out of that high school and I did not go back there in the fall of 1989. My mom was trying to find another school for me. This was a time of great stress for my mom and for me.

Fortunately I had enough sense not to turn to drugs or alcohol to forget my problems. I didn't want to become a drug addict or an alcoholic. My mom stayed strong and listened to me throughout the whole ordeal.

I just couldn't go back to that high school; that was not an option. I wasn't eighteen then, and the law said that I had to be in school. This was just like when I was in the sixth grade. It wasn't that I didn't want to attend school. On the contrary, I really WANTED an education! I just couldn't deal with my peers anymore, and the anxiety. I knew that I had to continue my education, and I wanted to, but I didn't know how. Later my question would be answered.

Looking back, reflecting on that school, I really wonder if things could have been different. If I had been into sports, acted like a jerk, and hung out with the in crowd, would things have been different? I wonder, would I have been liked? Maybe, but that's a moot question now. I'm wondering now, did the students there intend to cause me such emotional distress? What did they have against me? If I saw them today I would like to ask them that.

I learned from my high school experiences that I shouldn't have kept silent. I kept silent for far too long with all the details of my anxiety. There was just too much pressure at that school. I was so glad to be out of there. The whole experience should not have happened. To find someone that you can talk to and that you can vent your feelings to is very important. I should have talked more to my mom and dad because they were very supportive. It was still not known at that time that I had the social anxiety disorder.

Somehow my mom discovered a correspondence school, a way to complete high school. This was when things were starting to look up. I wouldn't have to actually attend school, but I would get my high school diploma. We found the American School, which was based out of Chicago. This was accredited by The North Central Branch and the National Home Study Council. Therefore, in December of 1989 I enrolled in the American School.

I would get my books through the mail, as well as my grades and tests. There was a form I had to fill out for everything I sent to the school. I really enjoyed studying and I always wondered what book would be coming next. My first two courses were psychology and English, respectively. Little did I know then that ten years later, in 1999, I would have a college degree with a minor plus in psychology and a major in English.

In January of 1990, we rang in a new year and a new decade with hope. My enrollment in the correspondence school, the American School, was a definite turning point for me. It meant that there would be no more insults, put downs, laughs behind my back, and other foolishness. I went from nowhere to somewhere.

Also in early 1990 I stopped seeing the therapists that couldn't help me. I went back to the person who helped me the most, a local psychiatrist that helped me in 1985. He told me that I could go far. I still remember him saying this. This was very encouraging.

In April of 1990, after finally having the school situation resolved, my mom and dad thought I should have a vacation. I enjoyed watching professional wrestling on television but I always wanted to see it in person.

My mom got tickets for my dad and me to see Wresltemania 6 in Toronto, Canada. This big event was going to be held in the brand new Toronto Skydome. My dad and I had a lot of fun on this trip. We saw all the top wrestlers of that time. In the main event, Hulk Hogan lost his title to the Ultimate Warrior. I felt a little sad that Hulk Hogan lost, but overall, I enjoyed the wrestling card and the vacation.

Meanwhile, I was doing well in my other subjects in my correspondence school. Then in May of 1990, I started my very first part-time job. My psychiatrist said that I needed to be in a social situation. I was hired at a restaurant chain where I washed dishes and bussed tables.

Curiously, at this restaurant worked one of the girls who was at my high school. I really liked her and I asked her out, but she wouldn't go out with me. She was a cheerleader at my former high school. I think that she thought that I was a high school dropout. It was hard working with her. It gave me a lot of anxiety. In fact, I think that a lot of people at this restaurant did not believe me when I said that I was home schooled. They would say things like, "Yeah right." or, "Whatever," or "Get real."

Anyway, I was proving that I could be in a social situation. Each day was a struggle but I was able to do it.

I continued to study all through 1990 and 1991 and I continued to work hard at the restaurant although at times 1 did feel a lot of anxiety when I worked there. For example, one of the managers that I really liked was transferred to another restaurant in a different state. It was very difficult getting used to new management. A person with anxiety disorder does not like a lot of change. I am a person who needs a stable environment no matter where I am. Change can be very difficult for a person with social anxiety disorder.

There were people at this restaurant who were very hard to work with. I was able to do it though. It was very difficult. I got through it with medication, deep breathing, and encouragement from my grandmother and my mom and dad.

Sometimes, if we could afford it, we would go to a baseball game. This was fun and I didn't feel too much anxiety. I was a little nervous being around the big crowds at the baseball games, but overall, I had a good time.

In February of 1991, my grandmother died, which was hard for my mom and for me. Although, my grandma did know that I was on the right track and that eventually I would graduate from high school. This was a major thing. At least grandma died knowing that things were getting better for us.

On April 23rd, 1991, I passed my driver's test. I remembered that I had a lot of anxiety before, after, and during the test, but I did pass. This was a good omen of things to come.

The estate of my grandmother's was divided equally among my mom and my two uncles. With the money from my grandma's house, my mom bought a condo. I felt some anxiety moving to a new place, and it would take a while to get settled in, but it would prove to be a gorgeous home.

I sat in the basement and I was working on my last subject, journalism. I finally could see the light at the end of the tunnel. All the hard work finally paid off and I finished my final high school subject at the end of 1991. I actually made it through high school, by way of the correspondence home schooling. My years in grade school and high school were very stressful, but I found a way to get through them.

In February of 1992 I got my high school diploma in the mail. I was so glad. Then in May of 1992 my mom had a party for me at a local restaurant. We invited family and friends and everyone had a good time.

On June 20, 1992, I took the S.A. T. test and I scored high. I studied a great deal for this test and l was very happy when the test was over. Then I began to look into college.

CHAPTER THREE: THE COLLEGE YEARS

In the summer of 1992, I was getting serious about starting college. However, even in college I would experience a lot of anxiety, and there would be setbacks.

That summer, I was scheduled to hear an orientation of how to register for classes at Milwaukee Area Technical College, also Called M.A.T.C. It was scheduled for 9:00 a.m. and I overslept. This was the first setback, but I did reschedule and I attended the next meeting. I registered for three classes in the fall of 1992 and I also planned to continue working at the restaurant where I worked for over two and a half years at that time. Everything was coming together for me.

The first day of class I was very nervous. It had been about three years since I had set foot in a classroom and I was no longer seeing the psychiatrist.

On the first day of class, my English professor handed out a single sheet of paper and asked us each to explain how we first learned how to write. I was in my element. I should have realized then and there that I would have English as my major. Little did I know then that I would graduate with a writing intensive English major.

One day in my sociology class I was talking to another student and she asked me if I was working on the paper for next week. I was dumbfounded. I said that I didn't know that there was a paper due next week. The girl sitting next to me said that she didn't know that either. The first girl said that it was on the syllabus and the instructor told her that she wasn't going to mention it to the class. The instructor said she wanted to see if the class looked at the syllabus. I had my paper ready in time. One thing I learned from this class was to always look at the syllabus. It is as valuable as a compass is to a captain at sea, or a road map to a tourist in an unfamiliar city. I also learned the lesson that you and ONLY you are responsible for your own actions; no one else is going to hold your hand or give you a warning like in high school. In college you either make it or you don't. YOU have to be self-reliant. Also, you have to find out everything for yourself. Don't rely on advisors or anyone else.

I thought on my first day about how far away graduation seemed. Would I actually graduate college after all the strife and troubles it took to just get through grade school and high school?

I got a D in my first history exam, and then an F in my first sociology exam. At first I thought that maybe I should just quit and explore another path. However, my mom said that if I do think of quitting, I should sleep on it. So I slept on it and I went to class the next morning.

My first semester I met a girl who was in both my English and sociology classes. I really liked her but she was going out with this guy. I had two tickets to a Bryan Adams concert, and l thought I'd ask her anyway. Bryan Adams was playing at the arena downtown. I talked with this girl a lot. She told me she wanted to go to Alaska to live with her dad. I really liked her and I knew that she had a boyfriend, but I asked her if she wanted to go to the Bryan Adams concert with me. She said yes. I picked her up that night and we had a great time.

Bryan Adams played all his hits and the place rocked. He was awesome. The opening act was great too. I asked the girl if it was too loud for her and she said it wasn't. After the concert the girl thanked me for a good time and I gave her a hug. A few days later I drove this girl home after our sociology class was cancelled. On the way home she told me that her boyfriend was out drinking the night we were at the concert and he drove home drunk. I guess that he thought I was trying to take her away from him, even though that wasn't my intention. Although I have to admit I did care for her. When the semester ended, we both went our separate ways.

In December of 1992, during the last week of classes for that semester, my sociology teacher said that she had no reason to pass me.

I talked with her for quite a while, and I asked her if there was anything that I could do to keep from failing the course. I really studied hard for the final exam, in hopes of not getting a failing grade for the course. The instructor also said to three other students that day that she had no reason to pass them. One of her students said that her tests should be matching and multiple choice. Then the instructor said to that student, "If we were at U.W.M. we wouldn't be having this conversation." In the end, I did pass the course and then I started preparing for my second semester in college. I was really relieved to have passed the course.

On November 28th, 1992, I had to quit my job at the restaurant where I worked. It was just too hard to study and work, plus trying to deal with all the anxiety. I gave the restaurant where I worked two weeks notice and we parted on good terms. It was either work at the restaurant or go to college. The stress of the anxiety prevented me from doing both.

On the essay portion of the final exam in English, I got an A. I scored fifty out of fifty possible points. My English teacher was impressed with my essay and he said that I must have known something about the subject to have written such a spectacular essay on the exam. It made me feel good to hear a compliment like that from an instructor, especially since the instructors at my grade school were always cutting down the kids and criticizing them. We were given this question: should gambling be limited in our state? I wrote nearly three pages and my English instructor wrote on my essay, "A very good attempt to bring in other sources." My first semester in college ended on a positive note, but I knew I still had my work cut out for me, and I still didn't know why I was so nervous all the time.

The spring semester of 1993 was a mixed bag. Once again, I missed quite a few classes due to the anxiety, and at one point my teacher asked me, a little worried, "Are you dropping out?" I told her that I wasn't and that I would make every effort to come more often. This really worried me because I wanted to pursue my college education and I enjoyed reading American literature, which was one of my classes that semester. I knew that I had to just force myself to get to class, even though it made me extremely nervous and uncomfortable. I wanted a college degree and nothing would stand in my way. I took deep breaths, prayed to the Lord, and I was able to get to class, but it wasn't easy.

There was an amazing difference between my grade school teachers and my college teachers. The college teachers were more caring. They were true professionals.

I thought that psychology would be interesting because I liked helping people so I took introduction to psychology in the summer of 1993. I had a very good instructor. I was able to get through the summer courses with relative ease, (I didn't feel a lot of anxiety and I studied hard and received good grades.) And I was preparing for the fall 1993 semester.

During the fall of 1993, during my child psychology class, I had a major problem. I had a panic attack. I would get these panic attacks from time to time, sometimes walking in the mall I would get very short of breath and my palms would get sweaty. Then I would have to leave the mall, or wherever I was because being there made me too nervous. One day in the child psychology class we were all supposed to get in groups. I didn't like doing this because it would make me very nervous.

We were supposed to get into groups to discuss something, and then one person was supposed to read the observations out loud to the class. No one wanted to read out loud and I sort of got stuck with it. During that reading all of a sudden I got very short of breath and my muscles tensed up. This was a bad experience that I still can vividly remember. Similar occurrences would happen when I walked into the class. I remember feeling this way during my high school years before I left my high school and enrolled in the American Correspondence School. I knew that I felt this way before and that it was more than just some "jitters" or normal anxiety that everyone experiences. This was the incident that led me once again to seek professional help. I was twenty years old at that time.

I was diagnosed with social anxiety disorder in September of 1993. It is difficult to explain this to certain people because some people would say, "Everyone gets nervous sometimes." Although that's true, it doesn't explain why some people get more nervous than others. Here is an example that I came up with: In comparing the social anxiety disorder to normal nervousness I will use another disorder such as comparing Alzheimer's Disease to normal forgetfulness. Normal forgetfulness would be when you forget your car keys. Alzheimer's Disease is when you forget that you OWN a car. Similarly, normal nervousness is when you get nervous speaking in front of a huge auditorium. Social Anxiety Disorder is when you CAN'T EVEN GO INTO the auditorium.

The social anxiety disorder is something that I have to live with and I have accepted this fact. The medicine that I currently take does help to some extent. This type of anxiety is caused by a chemical imbalance in the brain. Some people have a hard time understanding that what I have is not just normal nervousness, but an actual anxiety that help is needed to control.

On the day that I came back home from my child psychology class, I wanted to quit college altogether. I remember taking a chair up to my room, and sitting in it and really feeling down. Here again, the anxiety disorder was a real roadblock. I wanted to get to class but I just couldn't. I talked with my mom about it that day, and I wanted to continue school. Again I knew that I couldn't let anything stand in my way of getting a college degree. I would take deep breaths, pray, and try to get through it. I decided to drop that course and I took it at a later time. This would prove to be a wise decision since I met a professor who would prove to be very beneficial to me.

One of my psychology professors wrote me a letter that I received in January of 1994. It included my final exam and a letter: "Greetings, I trust that your mid semester break will afford you the opportunity for rest and recreation. Please know that I have enjoyed your presence in class. Surely, quality education can only take place when people like yourself are willing to invest time and take pride in the pursuit of personal excellence. Again, I have enjoyed our semester together."

It was nice of the professor to take time to write a letter like that. He was an excellent instructor. The instructors in college would prove to be infinitely better than the ones I had in grade school and high school. There was a world of difference; it was like night and day.

In the spring of 1994 I decided that I wanted to pursue psychology and I took only psychology subjects.

I remember driving to school hearing, "Rock Around The Clock" by Bill Haley and I thought to myself, "Man, rock has come a long way since then." In the same way, I had come a long way since grade school.

In the fall of 1994 once again the anxiety was getting to me and I remember thinking that I wanted to quit college. I didn't though, and I'm really glad now that I didn't.

I spoke with my child psychology teacher about my aspirations of transferring to a really good university. He suggested that I talk to the admissions office at Marquette University. You see, he taught part time at Marquette. I said that I would consider it. He said to at least talk to them, and the worst they could do was say no. I told him how good my grades were, and how much I studied, and he said that I should definitely talk to them.

There was another small setback, however. I ended up missing the final exam in child psychology because I had the stomach flu. Ironically, I had to go to Marquette University to take the final exam because that's where the professor had his main office. He told me to, "Look for the building with the funny shaped windows." So I went to Marquette, took the exam, and passed with flying colors. Little did I know when I took the exam that day that I would graduate from this prestigious university!

I had planned for a long time to see Wrestle mania 10, which was going to be held in New York City in 1994. My mom and I saved money so that I could fly out to Boston where I met my two friends. We drove from Boston to New York City and we stayed overnight in Stamford, Connecticut. This was a treat, but even during this vacation I felt some anxiety and I was taking medication. I enjoyed talking with my pals. We saw all the top tourist attractions of New York. I was amazed by the enormity of the city. Living in the midwest, I always viewed Chicago as a huge "big time" city, but arriving in New York City, I knew that even Chicago couldn't compare to New York. I never saw so many taxis in one place in my life. It was fun to have a change in atmosphere and experience a new setting, and it was a little intimidating as well. Visiting New York City was one of the best vacations that I ever had, and someday if I ever have the money I would most definitely go back. The professional wrestling event was held in Madison Square Garden. I also enjoyed seeing the Statue of Liberty, the Empire State Building, and many other historic parts of New York. Just to be in a city with such great diversity was an experience and an education in itself.

Back home, it was December of 1994 and my mom and I went into Marquette University to the admissions office. I was told that my grades were good and I knew I was in! I was accepted for the spring 1995 semester. My mom and I left the office and when we were in the hallway of Marquette Hall we were literally jumping for joy. I vowed that I would study hard and my instructors from M.A.T.C. the junior college wished me luck.

This was a huge turning point for my college career. I registered for classes and I was ready to take on anything, including the anxiety, to get my college degree. It took me about two hours to get my books since everyone in the university was getting their books that day. The lines at the bookstore were always very long on the first two days of class.

On January 19, 1995 I attended my first class at Marquette University. The class let out early and I went home and studied. At first I was a little intimidated attending such a big university. However, I studied my heart out and I got good grades my first semester. I knew I had arrived at the big time!

I still had to cope with the anxiety, but I was able to deal with it. I still felt nervous in class and l didn't like having to get in groups, but I wasn't going to let that or anything else stand in my way. Again, I coped with my anxiety by taking deep breaths, and praying.

In the fall of 1995 I hit another road block. I had virtually no computer experience whatsoever, and I felt very nervous when I went in the computer room at Marquette. I had a hard time getting my e-mail from the computer. I thought to myself, "I can't be beaten by a computer." Again I felt like quitting college, but I didn't. I hung in there. I was able to work the computer. Another obstacle was overcome. This was a rough semester, but I continued to study and I acquired a lot of knowledge.

Since then, I was able to get enough money together to buy a computer and today I am able to work a computer with relative ease. However, I still am not certain how to perform certain tasks on the computer. I still have a ways to go yet, but I'm getting there.

Now, the reader is probably thinking, how could someone let something like a computer make him want to quit college? This is a legitimate question. It really shouldn't be that big of a deal, should it? To many people it wouldn't be, however, with social anxiety disorder, when you are too nervous to get help from the information desk, and you are sitting there and struggling with something that you don't know how to work, it is pretty tough. It makes a person feel uncomfortable. I struggled and I felt like I had to get out of there. I'm glad that I overcame my anxiety and went back to the computer because today I don't know what I would do without my computer, especially since I am trying to pursue a career as a writer.

As autumn once again approached, I would get that feeling of not wanting to return to school. I got the shortness of breath, the sick to my stomach feeling, the sweaty palms, and the general feeling of nervousness. This happened every autumn, even when I was taking medication.

The fall of 1996 semester was a bad one. I was required to take a statistics course for my major of psychology, but I dropped it a few weeks into the semester. I still felt a great deal of anxiety and my grades were slumping, ending the year.

My mom and I were able to save enough money to go back down to Florida for a much needed vacation for the both of us. It was a cold Wisconsin winter and we enjoyed the "sunshine state."

When my mom and I got back to our house there was a letter from Marquette University in our mailbox. It was January 8th, 1997 and I got a letter from the university saying that if my grades did not improve during the next semester I would be required to withdraw. This worried me. The pressure was really on me to do well in my courses. I had come so far and I didn't want to blow it. I knew it was do or die. I was placed on probation and I had to meet with my advisor every week which was a real drag.

On April 13th, 1997, with all the stress, I got a bad cold. I was really afraid that I would be let go from the school, and I had worked so hard to get there. I just could not let that happen, I studied even more and I spent more time at the library, all in an effort to stay at Marquette. I still have many of the essays and papers that I turned in at Marquette. I studied hard and I spent a lot of time writing those papers. At the end of the semester, in May of 1997, I took the final exams and when I was finished I hoped and prayed that I had scored high enough on them so that I could stay at Marquette and not be required to withdraw.

I eventually received a letter stating that my grades were sufficient and I would be taken off of probation. All my studying had paid off. I was thankful and I breathed a sigh of relief. I also said a prayer of thanks. It was a huge relief, being able to stay at Marquette University.

That summer I once again took on statistics. Again I withdrew in a few days because it was too difficult. I never had a mind for math, but I knew that I had to take this course. It was very difficult for me. This was another roadblock.

One day, during the fall 1997 semester I looked outside and I saw the cold winds blowing and the brittle leaves falling. I started to wonder if I would ever graduate. Here again I felt discouraged and I wanted to quit, but I didn't.

I began 1998 with three psychology classes. This was the fourth time I started statistics.

This time I got a tutor and I still couldn't get it. So I dropped statistics for the fourth and final time and I changed my major from psychology to English. I had a tough time making this decision, but I decided that it was in my best interests to no longer pursue a degree in psychology; I wanted to go with my strength, which was, and still is, English. I don't regret taking all the psychology courses that I did. It helped me to tune in to other people and to communicate with other people. I learned a lot about why people do what they do and why they make the decisions they make. For example, why did the wise guys always accuse others of being wise guys? The answer is that they couldn't handle the fact that they were the wise guys so they had to project that behavior to somebody else. Now if I hadn't taken all the psychology classes that I did, I wouldn't understand why people act the way they do.

A word of wisdom to anyone who wants to attend college: In college you have to be self reliant. In other words, don't rely on anyone else to tell you things. You have to find out things for yourself.

In the summer of 1998 I took an American literature class in which I was the only guy in the class. I was a little intimidated by this. I met an interesting girl in this class. Her name was A.J. She wanted to concentrate on her career and I understood that. I really wanted a relationship with her but she was incredibly busy. We were good friends. I concentrated on studying and keeping my anxiety under control. I took deep breaths and I tried to relax. I always felt better when I saw A.J. A.J. and the other young women in this class helped me to see that it's good to talk about things with people, and that it's okay for a man to show his feelings and open up to others. In this class I wrote an essay about my high school years and how miserable I was then. This was the first time I expressed this to anyone other than my family. I liked this smaller class; it made me relax. A.J. and I talked when we came out of class. She showed me how to work the computer at Marquette's Memorial Library. One day in the summer we went to the cafeteria together. I really enjoyed her company. She was very intelligent.

One day A.J. and I went to the library and we sat outside. She had a cigarette since you aren't allowed to smoke inside the library. She told me that she had smoked since she was ten years old. She told me that she was never pregnant and that she never did drugs. One day I gave her a Guns N' Roses tape, and another day I gave her a Def Leppard tape. A.J. appreciated them and we were good friends. I was really hoping that this was the beginning of a relationship, but I guess it wasn't meant to be.

I took full time classes for the first time in the fall of 1998. Believe it or not, A.J the young lady I liked, was in three of my four classes! I was pleasantly surprised. I enjoyed seeing her in class every day.

I studied hard for my classes which included Shakespeare, History of the English Language, Chaucer, and Literature of the 16th century. In Shakespeare, we read all the famous plays including A Midsummer Night's Dream, King Lear, and Hamlet. The exams were all in an essay format, which I liked because I like writing. I devoted all of my time to studying and I ended the semester with good grades. It was fun reading Chaucer's "The Canterbury Tales" among other works. In one of my other classes, Literature of the 16th century, I was required to give a presentation, as was everybody, on a subject that was related to what we were studying. I was very nervous and I tried to put off this presentation as long as I possibly could. However, once again, I knew that this was something that I had to do if I wanted to graduate. I wouldn't let anything stand in my way of getting my college degree. I practiced the presentation for my mom several times. Luckily, we did not have to give it from memory. Occasionally in grade school there were times when I would have to give presentations by memory and this was really tough, not because of what I had to remember, but because of my anxiety. However, I was able to get through it in grade school, and I knew that I could do this presentation in college. I said a few prayers and took some deep breaths on the days leading up to the presentation day. I gave the presentation and 1 received a "B" which wasn't bad. I was satisfied with that. Another obstacle had been overcome. Another hurdle had been leaped and I was getting ready for the spring 1999 semester, my last semester in college.

Then in January of 1999 I started working at another restaurant, this time a local restaurant, not a national chain, I found out that I had to really hustle at this particular job, much like when I was at the other restaurant. Working and exercising is another good way to get rid of some anxiety and stress. I was able to lose a lot of weight and I felt a lot better when I did.

There was a worker at this restaurant who was very hard to get along with. Others complained about her, but yet the management didn't do anything about this worker. I tried to ignore this person, which worked to some extent. This person was a very hostile person, and with my studying of psychology I was able to deal with this individual.

Now I had just one subject left to become a Marquette University graduate. I couldn't believe it. I was not going to let anything stand in my way. My final subject was a course on Robert Frost. 1 studied Frost's work with a lot of passion and at the same time I worked washing dishes at the restaurant. Now I knew that nothing, absolutely nothing would stand in my way of becoming a Marquette University graduate.

I would still feel a lot of anxiety in this class and I had my ways of dealing with it. The deep breathing and telling myself that I could get through this helped. I dealt with the anxiety up to the very last days of college.

When I came out of my Robert Frost class, A.J. was waiting to come into the next class. I was glad that I could see her again, even if it was just for a few minutes. On May 5th, 1999, I saw her for the last time. She told me that she would graduate in August of that year, after only three years. One of the last times that I saw her she looked very pretty. She was wearing a gorgeous white dress. The final time I saw her we talked, held each others hand for a second, as if to say goodbye, and then I left for home.

It was time to put all my energy into studying for the final Exam in my Robert Frost class. I took a lot of time and I studied hard for the final exam, and the day finally came when I was officially finished with college. I took a deep breath of relief and said a prayer of thanks to God. It was on May 18th, 1999 that I found out for certain that I would graduate from Marquette University. All of the anxiety, anguish, and studying would finally pay off. In my living room I had a countdown sign that said, "23 days to graduation." Each day I would take down a page. In order to get the best possible grade I could I had to resign from the restaurant where I worked, and since I knew that I would be getting another job, a higher paying job, I wouldn't need to wash dishes anymore.

All the studying was finally over and all the preparations for graduation had to be made. I invited a lot of people. I had scrubbed all the floors in my house and I dusted everything. I wanted the house looking nice. My mom was too busy working so I took care of everything at home. My mom still works at a nursing home where there is a lot of stress, and we both hope that she can retire soon. My mom made the day memorable, and my dad did too. It was time to bask in the glory of the moment.

I awoke at 6:30 a.m. on May 23rd, 1999. The graduation ceremony took place in the Bradley Center in downtown Milwaukee. In the Bradley Center there were several speakers. I felt quite nervous, but happy at the same time. One girl gave a good speech comparing college to grocery shopping. She pointed out that no one has a perfect shopping experience, which is true. I thought that this was a good analogy. Then I spotted my mom and dad. They were up about ten rows to my right. There were some people during the ceremony that sprayed each other with silly glue and one person even had a beach ball and was tossing it around. There was no doubt about it. The big day had finally arrived.

When the dean confirmed the degrees everyone shouted for joy. This was by far the most dramatic moment of the entire ceremony. This was the actual moment of graduation: when we turned the tassels on our caps to the other side. It was an awesome day that I still haven't forgotten. A lot of flashbulbs went off. When the time came to march out I was elated, but I was a little disappointed that the ceremony was over. However, the party would begin at my house and I was looking forward to it.

The party started off with a bang and I was glad to have graduated. However, one thing put a damper on an otherwise happy day. My uncle Bob, who I was very close to and who my mom and I had gone with on vacations to the Wisconsin Dells, was taking chemotherapy, but made the effort to come to my party that day. My uncle got sick during the party and he had to be taken to the hospital. I felt very sad. My uncle had cancer in the form of lymphoma. At least my uncle did see that I graduated from college, though. I felt bad to see him so sick because he did so much for me and for other people.

On May 28th, 1999, my college degree came in the mail. I could have gone up on stage to get it, but I was too nervous and instead I requested that my degree be mailed to me. My mom gave me a poem for my graduation, and we still have it hanging in the living room. I put together a graduation photo album and I am still thankful that I graduated college. Nobody can ever take my college degree from me.

CHAPTER FOUR: THE YEARS AFTER COLLEGE

After I graduated it was time to test myself in the "real world." I thought about graduate school, but I owed so much money in student loans that I wanted to find work quickly. I found out that having a college degree in English was not as beneficial as I had thought it would be as far as getting work. The bills were piling up and I still didn't have much of a cash flow coming in. With the exception of my mom, I had virtually no income.

With the average price of a school textbook at forty, fifty, or even sixty dollars, credit card bills were starting to add up. It is my advice to anyone getting ready for college that you should not even apply for a credit card. It is too easy to get yourself into a large amount of debt. While attending school, in particular, college, you have to spend the majority of your time studying and attending classes. There is little time to work, and when you do work in college it is not at a high paying job. Therefore it is very easy to fall into a financial trap, by going far into debt.

I began attending Carroll College in Waukesha, Wisconsin in the autumn of 1999, and I also started a sales job at southridge mall which is near my home. This job was at a department store at southridge mall. It was not a good paying job, believe me. In the interview, I was asked, "Why should we hire you rather than a person with sales experience?" When you are interviewing for a job you really have to do your homework. This question sort of threw me a little bit. Especially with my anxiety I didn't think I did well. I was a little disappointed that they would rather have someone with sales experience than a Marquette University graduate. However, I did get the position. When you interview you have to try to be relaxed and confident, but not overconfident. Having social anxiety disorder, I really get uncomfortable during interviews and I think that is the reason why I've done poorly in some interviews. However, despite how difficult interviews might be, a person, even with anxiety, is able to be successful. I have to admit that in a fast paced environment I sometimes get overwhelmed and I cannot do well. I ended up not being able to stay at the job at the mall.

I withdrew from Carroll College because they didn't have the program that I needed. Also, I thought that it would take too long to get a Masters Degree and a P.H.D. degree. I looked at the amount of money that English teachers make and I realized that it wasn't enough to justify going further into debt, and taking all of that time. A professor of English at Marquette University helped me to make the decision. He said two years for a Masters and five years for a P.H.D. is a lot of time out of a person's life and a lot of money.

So then I tried to find work at an electronics store in the fall of 2000. I was hired and I worked there for a short time. I couldn't continue there because it was too stressful for a person that has anxiety disorder to the extent that I have it. I didn't like having to try to sell people what they didn't really need, which is something that this store wanted me to do. I would really get nervous at this store and I just couldn't stay there anymore.

I have found that it really is tough trying to get a good paying job after a person gets out of college. A person shouldn't have to look as hard as I have in order to find a decent paying job. Schools also should help steer students in the right direction. I am not just talking about colleges here. I believe that the whole system needs to be changed. The grade schools need to start incorporating a career class that shows the kids that they need to think about what they want to do with their lives from an early age. This course would also tell kids what training and or education they would need for any given career. For example, kids would know that for psychology they would need to do well in math. Also, in the case of a student who likes writing and English, he or she should be told that if you go on to get a college degree in English there is very little else that you can do with that degree besides teach English, which is something that I didn't really want to do. Also, there should be requirements that schools enlist people from all different careers to come in and talk to kids in grade school and high school to give them an idea of what they do for a living. I think that the schools all over need to do more to help their students. I also think that teachers should get much more money than they get for the hard work that they do.

I am now looking at the future with a little uncertainty. I have a college degree and I'm happy to be able to say that. As for a place of work I'm hoping that something will come through soon. In the meantime I have been doing a lot of writing. I have written over 800 poems and I am hoping to eventually get some of them published. I now know how to get a copyright and I am always working on a new writing project. I'm comfortable using a computer now and 1 enjoy going online.

Writing is another way that I have found that I can relieve my anxiety. I enjoy writing a lot and it also helps me to get rid of some of my "nervous energy." People deal with anxiety in many different ways. I have found that walking, running, or jogging, taking deep breaths, and praying to the Lord, as well as going to church, have helped me to lessen my anxiety. Medication has also helped me. Some people may find therapy very useful. The right doctor and the right medicine are very important. You have to find a doctor who cares and a therapist who is qualified.

There are many ways to get rid of anxiety and I hope that by reading this book people have been helped. I have tried to give some examples and tools throughout this book that can be of help for people who suffer from social anxiety disorder. Social anxiety and depression are very serious conditions which need medical attention and need to be understood by others. If you have a great mom and dad like I do, then you can talk to them. It is never a good idea to keep anything bottled up inside of you. Many times it helps to speak with a parent, family friend, clergyman, doctor, or social worker.

Although I have had a lot of strife with the anxiety in my life, every day I have managed to handle it and every day I look at as a new day that I have to try to make the most of.

Social anxiety disorder is similar to alcoholism because neither one ever goes away. It is not something that can be dismissed by rational thought, and it is not something that can be changed. An alcoholic must live the rest of his or her life with the struggle of not drinking. It is a day to day struggle that is certainly not easy. A person with anxiety disorder must live his or her life day to day dealing with the anxiety. It is thought that with age, the anxiety does decrease.

As we have seen in this book, there are many ways that I have battled with and dealt with my anxiety disorder. This book is meant to be that ray of hope for the person who cannot leave his or her residence. If this book can be found on the internet by him or her, and it is a source of help, then I have achieved a major goal.

I'm certain that other people with this problem will find this book helpful and those who don't will find it to be a way of understanding people who do have social anxiety disorder. Many Americans suffer from this and those who don't should be patient with those of us who do, and try to understand.

I feel that I have come a long way from my days in high school and grade school. I don't even seem or feel like the same person that I was then. I have matured and I have found out about relationships. I have visited some of the United States and I am very fortunate in that respect. I don't live in poverty. Other than the anxiety, I am in good health. I took on college and graduated. I did not let the anxiety hold me back from doing anything. I was able to find work and I know that I will again. The anxiety will not prevent me from working. I learned how to drive a car and even though I felt a lot of anxiety when I first started I learned the "rules of the road." I have many things working for me and I also have a great mom and dad and a nice place to live. I guess what I'm saying is that I am thankful for all that I have, and if I have to suffer through a lot of anxiety I know that a lot of people have things worse and that I have no reason to complain.

I think that we are moving towards the day when regular medical doctors can treat anxiety disorder and depression. These disorders are serious, but do not prevent a person from thinking rationally.

There are still some days, even today, when I find that it is somewhat difficult to go in a grocery store or a shopping center alone. It seems that it helps my anxiety when there is someone with me. This is further proof that the anxiety does not completely go away.

This book was intended to be a helpful source in understanding social anxiety disorder. It is by no means meant to be a replacement for therapy or medication when needed. With deep breathing exercises as well as proper medication, a person with this disorder can lead a better life. Hopefully the trials and tribulations that I experienced can be used to help others.

Even though at times things looked very bleak for me I refused to give up. Even with the anxiety I found a way to continue. I know that it can be managed. I control it; it does not control me. Perhaps someday there will be an even better medicine that will make people like me completely at ease in society. My advice to anyone, whether they have anxiety or not is to pursue your goal until you reach it.

THE END

ABOUT THE AUTHOR

Mark Pagel, the author of, *Growing Up With Anxiety Disorder*, is well-versed in writing, and has a degree in English-Writing Intensive from Marquette University, along with a minor plus in Psychology.

The author was first printed at age seventeen, and has had letters printed in the *Milwaukee Journal Sentinel* and the *Chicago Tribune*.

He has experienced firsthand the anxieties which school can present, especially when one has a disorder of this nature.

www.ingramcontent.com/pod-product-compliance
Lightning Source LLC
Chambersburg PA
CBHW051429280526
45785CB00003B/1221